Osteoporosis Diet

and

Exercises

"Bones of Bliss: Nourishing Your Way to Radiant Health"

ANNE FINLEY

Copyright © 2024

All Rights Are Reserved

The content in this book may not be reproduced, duplicated, or transferred without the express written permission of the author or publisher. Under no circumstances will the publisher or author be held liable or legally responsible for any losses, expenditures, or damages incurred directly or indirectly as a consequence of the information included in this book.

Legal Remarks

Copyright protection applies to this publication. It is only intended for personal use. No piece of this work may be modified, distributed, sold, quoted, or paraphrased without the author's or publisher's consent.

Disclaimer Statement

Please keep in mind that the contents of this booklet are meant for educational and recreational purposes. Every effort has been made to offer accurate, up-to-date, reliable, and thorough information. There are, however, no stated or implied assurances of any kind. Readers understand that the author is providing competent counsel. The content in this book originates from several sources. Please seek the opinion of a competent professional before using any of the tactics outlined in this book. By reading this book, the reader agrees that the author will not be held accountable for any direct or indirect damages resulting from the use of the information contained therein, including, but not limited to, errors, omissions, or inaccuracies.

TABLE OF CONTENTS

INTRODUCTION

Greetings from a journey that touches on the core of your wellbeing and goes beyond the pages of this book. Armed with three decades of publishing experience, a dedication to your vitality, and a passion for enabling you to take charge of your own health narrative, we set out on a revolutionary investigation of the realm of bone health with "Osteoporosis Diet and Exercises." We explore the complex picture of osteoporosis in the first few chapters. This is a disease that is frequently ignored until it starts to interfere with daily life. Osteoporosis is defined not just by weakening bones but also by a call to action. It is a journey we must travel together. We solve the enigmas around its origins, look at risk factors that could be imperceptibly harming you, and illuminate the subtle cues your body might be giving off.

The focus shifts to diet, the engine of bone health, as we go into Chapter 2. Consider your diet as a tactical toolkit to prevent osteoporosis rather than just a list of foods. We break down the vital nutrients that are important for strong bones and lead you through a carefully chosen list of foods that can serve as the foundation of your diet to prevent osteoporosis. Get ready for a taste experience as we share mouthwatering dishes and useful meal planning advice designed to strengthen your bones.

Your personal roadmap, found in Chapter Three, will help you create a personalized osteoporosis diet plan. We give you the freedom to customize your diet to match your own needs, preferences, and lifestyle—there are no one-size-fits-all answers here. Learn the skill of purposeful grocery shopping so that every item in your cart strengthens the inner fortress you are creating.

In Chapter Four, the story then deftly shifts to the realm of exercise. Imagine your body as a strong sculpture that is only waiting for the correct motions to mold it. We provide you with a safe and efficient program by demystifying the world of bone-density-enhancing activities. Our advice guarantees that your fitness path is in line with your bone health objectives, regardless of your level of experience or inexperience.

But this is a lifestyle guide, not just a book of numbers and data. Chapters Five through Seven examine a wider range of lifestyle modifications that are required for the best possible bone health. We provide you with the tools to cultivate an environment that supports healthy bones, from tackling bad behaviors like drinking and smoking to embracing the benefits of vitamin D from the sun.

As the book progresses, Chapter Eight incorporates true success stories that provide a compelling portrait of people who overcame osteoporosis in spite of all the difficulties. These tales are not only motivational but also uplifting, showing that anyone may begin a journey towards stronger bones with dedication and education.

Are you prepared to set out on this inspiring journey to healthy living and stronger bones? As we explore the possibilities for a life full of power and energy, let the pages that follow serve as your mentor, confidante, and inspiration. The path to ideal bone health starts right now.

CHAPTER ONE

OSTEOPOROSIS UNVEILED

Definition and Causes

Definition: Osteoporosis

A medical disorder called osteoporosis is defined by the weakening of bones, which makes them brittle and more prone to breaking. The translation of the term "osteoporosis" is "porous bones," emphasizing the loss of bone mass and density. Bone tissue normally regenerates continuously, with new bone growing in place of the old. This equilibrium is upset by osteoporosis, making bones porous, fragile, and prone to fractures, even in the case of minor damage.

Causes of Osteoporosis:

1. Age: Osteoporosis and aging are frequently linked. People's bone density naturally declines with age. This is especially true for women whose estrogen levels drop after menopause, which affects bone density.

2. Changes in Hormones: Hormonal abnormalities are a major contributor to osteoporosis. Bone loss is partly caused by decreased testosterone levels in men and decreased estrogen levels in women after menopause.

Factors may also include hormonal abnormalities, such as hyperthyroidism or diseases of the adrenal glands.

3. Inadequate nutritional support: Bone health can be harmed by an inadequate intake of some vital minerals, including calcium and vitamin D. The development and upkeep of strong bones depend on these nutrients. Osteoporosis may occur as a result of a diet deficient in these nutrients.

4. Generic Factors: Osteoporosis may be significantly influenced by family history. People may be more susceptible to osteoporosis if their family has a history of fractures or the disorder.

5. Lifestyle choices: There are lifestyle variables that increase one's risk of osteoporosis. Bone health can be adversely affected by smoking, excessive alcohol use, a sedentary lifestyle, and a lack of physical activity, particularly weight-bearing exercises.

6. Health Issues: The chance of developing osteoporosis can be raised by certain medical disorders and therapies. Bone density can be impacted by diseases such as rheumatoid arthritis, chronic renal disease, and hormone imbalances. Furthermore, prolonged use of some drugs, such as glucocorticoids, might exacerbate bone loss.

7. Low Body Weight and Body Mass Index (BMI): A lower body weight, or BMI, may result in less bone mass, which makes a person more susceptible to osteoporosis. This is particularly important when dealing with eating disorders or illnesses that interfere with the absorption of nutrients.

8. Race and ethnicity: The prevalence of osteoporosis varies among racial and ethnic groupings. People of Asian or Caucasian heritage, for instance, might be more at risk than people of African heritage.

Risk Factors

Several risk factors contribute to the development of osteoporosis, increasing the likelihood of bone loss and fractures. It's essential to be aware of these factors to take preventive measures and manage potential risks. Here are some key risk factors associated with osteoporosis:

1. Age: Osteoporosis is more common as people age, especially in elderly men and women who have gone through menopause. As people age, their bone density gradually decreases, increasing the risk of fractures.

2. Gender: In general, women are more likely than men to acquire osteoporosis. This is particularly true when estrogen levels drop after menopause, hastening the loss of bone.

3. Changes in Hormones: Bone loss can be exacerbated by hormonal abnormalities, such as those brought on by menopause or other medical disorders. An elevated risk of osteoporosis is linked to low testosterone levels in males and low estrogen levels in women.

4. Family History: A hereditary propensity to osteoporosis or fractures may be indicated by a family history of the disorder. A person may be more susceptible if their parents or siblings had fractures caused by osteoporosis.

5. Low BMI and Body Weight: People who are underweight or have a low body mass index (BMI) may have less bone mass, which increases their risk of developing osteoporosis. This is especially important for people with eating problems or illnesses that interfere with the absorption of nutrients.

6. Inadequate Nutritional Support: Bone health can be harmed by inadequate consumption of certain nutrients, particularly calcium and vitamin D. The risk of osteoporosis is increased with a diet deficient in certain nutrients.

7. Lifestyle Factors: There are lifestyle decisions that increase the risk of osteoporosis. Smoking, binge drinking, and a lack of physical activity, particularly weight-bearing exercises, can all have a detrimental effect on bone density.

8. Medical Conditions: Long-term illnesses that affect the kidneys, rheumatoid arthritis, and hormonal imbalances might raise the risk of osteoporosis. Furthermore, long-term use of some drugs, such as glucocorticoids, might exacerbate bone loss.

9. Ethnicity and Race: The risk of osteoporosis can differ between racial and ethnic groupings. Compared to people of African heritage, those of Asian or Caucasian descent might be more at risk.

10. Previous Fractures: A history of fractures, particularly following minor trauma, may be an indication of impaired bone health and put one at greater risk of developing new fractures.

11. Low Physical Activity: Low levels of physical activity, especially weight-bearing activities that promote the growth of new bones, can lead to a decrease in bone density.

Signs and Symptoms

Osteoporosis is commonly known as a "silent disease" since it usually worsens without causing any symptoms until a fracture. Nonetheless, certain indications and symptoms could surface as the illness worsens. It's critical to be aware of these signs, particularly if you have osteoporosis risk factors. These are a few typical indications and symptoms:

Fractures: Fractures are frequently the most obvious indication of osteoporosis, especially those that occur in the hip, wrist, and spine. These fractures can occur with little to no force and are an important sign of weakening bones.

Height Loss: A progressive decrease in height can occur from compression fractures in the vertebrae of the spine caused by osteoporosis. This could result in a bent or stooped posture,known as kyphosis.

Back Pain: Chronic back pain can be brought on by compression fractures in the spine. Localized discomfort that gets worse when you move, sneeze, or cough.

Changes in Posture: Posture may noticeably alter following vertebral fractures, with the upper spine possibly curving forward.

Decreased Grip Strength: A decrease in grip strength may result from weakening of the hand and wrist bones.

Teeth loss and gum recession: A higher incidence of tooth loss and receding gums are two effects of osteoporosis on the jawbone.

Brittle Nails: It is possible to notice alterations in the strength and texture of nails, with brittleness increasing.

Difficulty Standing or Walking: Problems standing or walking can result from fractures in weight-bearing bones like the hip or pelvis.

General Weakness and Fatigue: All-around exhaustion and weakness can be attributed to physical limits brought on by fractures and chronic pain.

CHAPTER TWO

THE ROLE OF NUTRITION IN BONE HEALTH

Essential Nutrients for Strong Bones

A balanced diet that includes the different nutrients that support bone density, structure, and general health is necessary to maintain strong and healthy bones. The following nutrients are vital for healthy bones:

1. Calcium: Because it gives teeth and bones the structural support they require, calcium is an essential mineral for bone health. Good sources of calcium include dairy products, leafy greens, tofu, fortified plant-based milk, and some fish (including sardines and salmon).

2. Vitamin D: For calcium to be absorbed in the intestines and used in the creation of bones, vitamin D is essential. Good sources of vitamin D include sunshine, fortified dairy or plant-based milk, egg yolks, and fatty fish (such as salmon and mackerel).

3. Phosphorus:

Together with calcium, phosphorus helps to create and preserve bone structure. Foods, including dairy, meat, fish, nuts, and whole grains, contain it.

4. Magnesium: Magnesium is necessary to transform vitamin D into its active form and contribute to bone mineralization. Legumes, whole grains, nuts, seeds, and leafy green vegetables are foods high in magnesium.

5. Vitamin K: Vitamin K aids in calcium regulation in the bones and has a role in bone mineralization. Broccoli, Brussels sprouts, leafy green vegetables, and fermented foods are foods high in vitamin K.

6. Protein: Protein is an essential component that gives bones their strength and shape. Lean meats, poultry, fish, dairy products, eggs, legumes, and plant-based protein sources like tempeh and tofu are all excellent sources of protein.

7. Zinc: Zinc is necessary for the metabolism of bones and aids in the production of collagen, a protein that is vital to the health of bones. Meat, dairy products, nuts, seeds, and whole grains all contain it.

8. Copper: Copper aids in the production of collagen and preserves bone density. It can be found in foods such as whole grains, nuts, seeds, seafood, and organ meats.

9. Boron: By affecting the metabolism of calcium, magnesium, and vitamin D, boron promotes bone health.

Boron can be found in foods such as fruits, vegetables, nuts, and legumes.

10. Vitamin C: Collagen is a crucial component of bones and is produced by the body using vitamin C. Broccoli, bell peppers, strawberries, and citrus fruits are high in vitamin C.

Foods to Include in Your Osteoporosis Diet

A well-balanced diet rich in essential nutrients is crucial for promoting bone health and preventing osteoporosis. Here are some foods to include in your osteoporosis diet:

1. Dairy Products:

- Milk
- Yogurt
- Cheese
- Fortified plant-based milk alternatives (soy, almond, or oat milk)

2. Leafy Green Vegetables:

- Kale
- Spinach
- Swiss chard
- Collard greens

- Broccoli

3. Fatty Fish:

- Salmon
- Sardines
- Mackerel
- Trout

4. Fortified Foods:

- Fortified cereals
- Fortified plant-based milk alternatives
- Fortified orange juice

5. Tofu and Soy Products:

- Tofu
- Edamame
- Soybeans
- Soy milk

6. Nuts and Seeds:

- Almonds
- Sesame seeds
- Chia seeds
- Flaxseeds

7.Lean Proteins:

- Chicken
- Turkey
- Fish
- Lean cuts of beef or pork

8. Whole Grains:

- Quinoa
- Brown rice
- Oat Whole wheat

9. Legumes:

- Chickpeas
- Lentils
- Black beans
- Kidney beans

10. Fruits:

- Oranges
- Strawberries
- Pineapple
- Kiwi

11. Vegetables:

- Bell peppers
- Sweet potatoes

- Brussels sprouts
- Cabbage

12. Dried Fruits:

- Dried figs
- Apricots

13. Eggs:

Eggs are a good source of vitamin D and protein.

14. Lean Meats:

Lean cuts of meat, such as skinless poultry and lean beef, provide essential proteins and minerals.

15. Foods Rich in Omega-3 Fatty Acids:

- Walnuts
- Chia seeds
- Flaxseeds
- Fatty fish (salmon, mackerel)

Nutritional Supplements

1. Supplements for Calcium: One essential mineral for healthy bones is calcium. In the event that dietary consumption is inadequate, calcium supplements could be advised. For optimal absorption, it is usually recommended to take calcium supplements with meals.

Calcium supplements come in a variety of forms, including calcium citrate and carbonate.

2. Vitamin D Supplements: Calcium absorption in the intestines depends on vitamin D. Vitamin D is naturally found in sunlight, although supplements could be needed, particularly for people who don't get much sun exposure. The best type of vitamin D to take as a supplement is D3.

3. Magnesium Supplements: For the health of your bones, magnesium and calcium work together. Even though magnesium may be found in a wide variety of foods, some people may find that taking supplements can help, particularly if their diet is deficient.

4. Vitamin K Supplements: Bone mineralization is aided by vitamin K. While leafy green vegetables are a good source, people who have problems with absorption or limited dietary intake may want to think about taking supplements.

5. Omega-3 or Fish Oil Supplements: Omega-3 fatty acids, which are present in fish oil supplements, may support bone health and have anti-inflammatory properties. To find out the right dosage, speak with a medical practitioner.

6. Boron Supplements: A trace element called boron may help maintain the health of your bones. Although it can be found in some foods, people with poor dietary intake may want to think about taking supplements.

7. Collagen Supplements: A protein called collagen gives bones their structure. Supplemental collagen may help maintain bone health, but further studies are required to confirm this.

8. Protein Supplements: Since protein is essential for healthy bones, some people may require supplements, particularly if their diet isn't sufficiently high. Supplements, including plant-based protein, collagen protein, or whey protein, are possible choices.

CHAPTER THREE

CRAFTING YOUR OSTEOPOROSIS DIET PLAN

Customizing Your Diet Based on Needs

Customizing your diet to meet your unique demands is an essential part of managing osteoporosis. The factors that determine particular nutritional needs include age, gender, health conditions, dietary preferences, and lifestyle. The following recommendations can help you tailor your osteoporosis diet:

One of the most important aspects of managing osteoporosis is adjusting your diet to your unique requirements. Certain nutritional requirements are influenced by a person's age, gender, health, food preferences, and way of life.

The following suggestions can assist you in customizing your diet for osteoporosis:

1. Intake of Calcium: Calculate your daily calcium requirements while taking possible supplements and food sources into account. It's critical to tailor calcium consumption because different people have different needs. Make sure you eat a variety of foods high in calcium, take supplements as needed, and keep an eye on your daily intake overall.

2. Vitamin D Levels: Use blood testing to determine your vitamin D levels. Your healthcare professional may suggest vitamin D supplements to achieve optimal levels based on your unique circumstances, dietary intake, and amount of sun exposure.

3. Protein Intake: Consider how much protein you consume, as it is necessary for strong bones. Make sure your diet includes both plant- and animal-based protein sources, and if your daily needs are not met, think about taking protein supplements.

4. Phosphorus and Magnesium Equilibrium: Adjust your diet so that the amounts of phosphorus and magnesium are balanced. Together with calcium, these minerals support healthy bones. Include foods high in magnesium and make sure your supplies of phosphorus are in balance.

5. Include Foods Rich in Vitamin K: Tailor your diet to include foods high in vitamin K, like leafy green vegetables. For the mineralization of bones and general bone health, vitamin K is essential.

6. Control Sodium Consumption: Watch how much salt you eat, since too much sodium might cause your urine to lose calcium. To help decrease salt levels, give whole, unprocessed foods priority and limit processed foods.

7. Stay Hydrated: Sufficient hydration is necessary for good health in general, including healthy bones. Adjust your fluid intake to suit your specific demands, taking age, level of physical activity, and climate into account.

8. Monitor and adjust: Keep a close eye on your nutrition and bone health. Modify your diet plan as necessary to account for changes in exercise levels, dietary preferences, or health.

9. Incorporate Lifestyle Factors: Tailor your diet to a lifestyle that is healthy for your bones. Take up weight-bearing activities, give up smoking, drink less alcohol, and make sure you get enough sunlight exposure to synthesize vitamin D.

Meal Planning and Recipes

Meal planning is a crucial aspect of maintaining a balanced diet that supports bone health in individuals with osteoporosis. Here's a sample meal plan along with recipes that incorporate nutrients essential for strong bones:

Sample Meal Plan:

Breakfast:

Greek Yogurt Parfait:

 Ingredients:

1 cup Greek yogurt (high in calcium and protein) 1/2 cup granola (fortified with calcium and vitamin D) Mixed berries (rich in vitamin C for collagen synthesis) Drizzle of honey (optional)

Lunch:

Salmon and Quinoa Salad:

Ingredients:

Grilled or baked salmon (rich in omega-3 fatty acids and vitamin D)

Quinoa (a good source of protein and magnesium) Spinach or kale (high in calcium)

Cherry tomatoes and cucumber Lemon vinaigrette dressing

Snack:

Almond and Dried Fruit Mix:

Ingredients:

Almonds (rich in calcium and magnesium)
Dried figs and apricots (good sources of calcium and boron)

Dinner:

Vegetarian Stir-Fry with Tofu:

Ingredients:

Tofu (plant-based protein and calcium)
Broccoli, bell peppers, and bok choy (vegetables rich in vitamin K and calcium)

Brown rice (whole grain for phosphorus)
Sesame seeds for garnish

Recipes:

1. Greek Yogurt Parfait:

Layer Greek yogurt with granola and mixed berries in a glass.

Repeat layers until the glass is filled. Drizzle with honey if desired.

This parfait provides a calcium- and protein-packed start to the day.

2. Salmon and Quinoa Salad:

Grill or bake salmon until cooked. Cook the quinoa according to the package instructions.

In a bowl, combine cooked quinoa, flaked salmon, chopped spinach or kale, cherry tomatoes, and cucumber.

Drizzle with a lemon vinaigrette dressing made with olive oil, lemon juice, Dijon mustard, salt, and pepper.

3. Almond and Dried Fruit Mix:

Combine almonds, dried figs, and dried apricots in a snack-sized bowl.

This mix offers a blend of calcium, magnesium, and boron.

4. Vegetarian Stir-Fry with Tofu: Press the tofu to remove excess water and cut it into cubes. In a wok or skillet, stir-fry tofu until golden brown. Add broccoli, bell peppers, and bok choy to the wok. Stir in a sauce made with soy sauce, ginger, garlic, and a touch of sesame oil.

Serve the stir-fry over brown rice and garnish with sesame seeds.

Tips for Grocery Shopping

Grocery shopping for osteoporosis involves selecting nutrient-dense foods that support bone health.

Here are some tips to make your grocery shopping trips bone-friendly:

1. Prioritize calcium-rich foods:

Include dairy products (or fortified plant-based alternatives), such as milk, yogurt, and cheese. Opt for calcium-fortified foods like fortified cereals, plant-based milk, and juices.

2. Choose leafy greens:

Load up on leafy green vegetables like kale, spinach, and collard greens. These are rich in calcium and other essential nutrients.

3. Pick Fatty Fish:

Choose fatty fish such as salmon, sardines, and mackerel. These provide omega-3 fatty acids and vitamin D, which are crucial for bone health.

4. Select lean proteins:

Opt for lean protein sources like chicken, turkey, fish, tofu, and legumes. Protein is vital for bone structure and maintenance.

5. Include Whole Grains:

Choose whole grains such as quinoa, brown rice, oats, and whole wheat bread. These provide phosphorus, magnesium, and other bone-supporting nutrients.

6. Add Nuts and Seeds:

Incorporate almonds, walnuts, chia seeds, and flaxseeds into your shopping list. These are rich in calcium, magnesium, and omega-3 fatty acids.

7. Get Your Vitamin K:

Include vegetables like broccoli, Brussels sprouts, and cabbage, which are high in vitamin K, essential for bone mineralization.

8. Explore Fortified Foods:

Look for fortified foods, including cereals, plant-based milk, and orange juice. These can contribute additional calcium and vitamin D to your diet.

9. Check labels for nutrient content:

When choosing packaged foods, read labels to check for calcium and vitamin D content. Select products that contribute to your daily nutritional needs.

10. Consider Supplements:

add supplements to your shopping list. Common supplements for osteoporosis may include calcium, vitamin D, and other nutrients.

11. Limit Sodium Intake:

Be mindful of processed and packaged foods, as they may be high in sodium. Excessive sodium intake can contribute to calcium loss.

12.Include fresh fruits:

Incorporate fruits like oranges, strawberries, and kiwi into your diet. These fruits provide vitamin C, which is important for collagen synthesis in bones.

13.Choose Low-Fat Dairy:

If you consume dairy, opt for low-fat or fat-free varieties to reduce your saturated fat intake.

14.Stay Hydrated:

Include water and low-calorie beverages in your shopping cart. Staying hydrated is essential for overall health, including bone health.

15. Plan Meals Ahead:

Plan your meals and create a shopping list to ensure you have a variety of bone-healthy foods available at home.

CHAPTER FOUR

EXERCISE FOR STRONG BONES

Types of Exercises Beneficial for Osteoporosis

Exercise is essential for managing osteoporosis because it keeps bone density intact, enhances balance, and lowers the chance of fractures. It is crucial to concentrate on weight-bearing and muscle-strengthening exercises when doing osteoporosis workouts.

1. Weight-Bearing Exercises:

- **Walking:** A straightforward and efficient weight-bearing activity that's easy to work into regular schedules.

- **Aerobic Dancing:** Dancing exercises can be entertaining and good for your bones.

- **Stair Climbing:** Accenting stairs strengthens the lower body and helps load the bones.

2. Strength Training:

- **Resistance Exercises:** Using weights or resistance bands improves bone strength by helping to develop and maintain muscle mass.

- **Bodyweight Exercises:** You can modify exercises like push-ups, lunges, and squats to meet your own fitness level.

3. Balance and Stability Exercises:

- **Tai Chi:** Enhance your flexibility and balance with this low-impact workout that includes deep breathing and slow, flowing motions.
- **Yoga:** Some yoga poses encourage flexibility and stability by emphasizing strength and balance.
- **Pilates:** Pilates movements focus on general body control, stability, and strength of the core.

4. Functional Exercises:

- **Functional Movements:** To improve functioning and lower the risk of falls, include exercises that imitate commonplace actions like bending, lifting, and reaching
- **Balance Exercises:** Practice balancing on uneven surfaces, walking heel to toe, or standing on one leg.

5. Flexibility and Range of Motion Exercises:

- **Stretching:** Perform dynamic and static stretches to maintain flexibility and increase joint range of motion.

- **Yoga and Pilates:** These exercises improve flexibility as well as balance.

6. Impact Activities:

- **Jumping Jacks:** Managed jumps create a regulated impact that promotes the growth of new bone.

- **Jumping Rope:** For bone health, a low-impact jumping rope can be beneficial.

7. Water-Based Activities:

- **Diving:** Swimming and water aerobics are low-impact activities that can enhance general fitness and are appropriate for individuals with joint difficulties, even though they do not require lifting weights.

8. Activities for Whole-Body Vibration:

- **Platforms for Whole-Body Vibration:** These gadgets vibrate, which may increase bone density by encouraging muscular contractions.

Creating a Safe and Effective Exercise Routine

A safe and efficient osteoporosis exercise program should include a range of weight-bearing, muscle-strengthening, balancing, and flexibility exercises. This is an example of a workout plan.

1. Warm-Up (5-10 Minutes)

Warming up the heart and muscles with light aerobic movement is known as the "cardiovascular warm-up. Examples include marching in place, stationary cycling, and brisk walking.

2. Joint Mobility Exercises: Mild motions to increase range of motion and warm up joints. Wrist flexor stretches, ankle rolls, and shoulder circles are a few examples.

20–30 Minute Weight-Bearing and Muscle-Strengthening Exercises:

3. Bodyweight Squats: Place your feet shoulder-width apart as you stand.

Bend down into a squat while maintaining your knees over your ankles. Perform between 10 and 15 repetitions.

4. Lunges: Step forward with one foot and bend both knees at that point.

Take a step back and exchange your legs. Work each leg for ten to fifteen repetitions.

5. Wall Push-Ups: Position yourself at arm's length in front of a wall. Place your hands shoulder-height on the wall.

Push-ups should be done with a straight body. Repeat ten to fifteen times.

6. Resistance Band Workouts: Use resistance bands in workouts such as leg presses, chest presses, and seated rows.

Adhere to a fitness expert's program created to focus on your main muscle groups.

 Exercises for Stability and Balance (10–15 minutes):

7. One-Leg Supports: If necessary, grasp onto a firm surface while standing on one leg. Switch legs, hold for another 20 to 30 seconds, then repeat.

8. The heel-to-toe walk: involves walking in a straight line while putting one foot's heel in front of the other's toes.

Take ten to fifteen steps.

9. Yoga or Tai Chi Poses: Include mild balancing poses like warrior or tree pose from tai chi or yoga.

Adhere to a regimen for beginners that emphasizes stability.

Stretching and Flexibility (5–10 minutes):

10. Dynamic Stretching: To improve flexibility and warm up muscles, perform dynamic stretches. Arm circles, leg swings, and torso twists are among the examples.

11. Static Stretching: Concentrate on the lower back, hips, thighs, and shoulders while holding static stretches for the main muscle groups.

Hold for 15 to 30 seconds after each stretch.

Relax for 5–10 minutes:

12. Slow Walking or Marching in Place: Lower the intensity gradually to return the heart rate to normal.

13. Deep Breathing and Relaxation: Use relaxation methods and deep breathing exercises to aid in healing and lessen tension.

Safety Tips:

Listen to Your Body:

If you experience pain or discomfort, modify or skip exercises as needed.

Use Proper Form:

Focus on proper technique to prevent injuries.

Progress Gradually:

Start with easier exercises and gradually increase intensity and duration over time.

Stay Hydrated:

Drink water throughout your exercise routine.

Include Variety:

Incorporate a mix of exercises to target different muscle groups and keep the routine engaging.

Incorporating Weight-Bearing and Resistance Exercises

For those with osteoporosis, maintaining and increasing bone density requires weight-bearing and resistance workouts. Here's how to include these kinds of workouts in your regimen:

Exercises with Weights:

1. Walking:

On most days of the week, begin with 30 minutes or more of vigorous walking.

Increase duration, speed, or intensity gradually over time. Make use of supportive walking shoes.

2. Stair Climbing: Include stair climbing in your daily exercise regimen. As you gain strength, start with a few flights and progressively increase.

3. Aerobic Dancing: Take part in aerobic dance sessions that don't require much movement. Select exercises that involve deliberate motions and stay away from abrupt leaps.

4. Elliptical Training: Employ an elliptical machine to work out while bearing weight in a low-impact manner. Pay attention to deliberate, fluid motions.

5. Hiking: Discover hiking paths for the benefits of weight-bearing exercise combined with cardiovascular fitness.

Select trails with different elevations for a greater challenge.

Resistance Exercises

Sixth, perform bodyweight squats. Place your feet shoulder-width apart.

Bend your knees so they are over your ankles to lower your body.

Do two sets of ten to fifteen repetitions.

7. Lunges: Take a single footstep forward and bend both knees to the side.

Perform two sets of ten to fifteen repetitions on each leg, switching legs.

8. Wall Push-Ups: Position yourself at arm's length in front of a wall.

Press-ups against the wall should be done in two sets of ten to fifteen repetitions.

9. Seated Leg Press: For seated leg press exercises, use resistance machines.

Change the weight and carry out 2 sets of 10 to 15 repetitions.

10. Bicep Curls: To perform bicep curls, use resistance bands or dumbbells.

completing two sets of 10 to 15 repetitions.

11. Seated Row: For seated row exercises, use resistance bands or a cable machine.

Perform 2 sets of 10–15 repetitions.

12. Calf Raises: Take a flat stance, raise yourself up to your toes, and then lower yourself back down. Complete two sets of 15 to 20 repetitions.

Advice on Including Exercises:

Progress Gradually: As your strength increases, progressively increase the weights and intensity.

Pay Attention to Form: To avoid injuries, perform exercises with the correct form.

Include Variety: Switch up your weight-bearing and resistance training routines to target different muscle groups.

Warm-up and cool-down: Prior to beginning resistance training, always warm up with some mild cardiovascular exercise.

Stretch after cooling down to increase suppleness and lessen soreness in the muscles.

Consistency is key. Aim for at least two days of resistance exercises each week, progressively increasing as fitness allows.

CHAPTER FIVE

LIFESTYLE CHANGES FOR BONE HEALTH

Smoking and Its Impact on Osteoporosis

Smoking negatively affects bone health and raises the possibility of fractures and osteoporosis. An outline of the effects of smoking on the skeletal system is provided here:

Smoking Effects on Bone Health:

1. Decreased Bone Density: One of the main factors influencing bone strength, bone mineral density (BMD), is correlated with smoking. Compared to non-smokers, smokers typically have lower bone mass.

2. Hormonal Imbalance: Smoking affects the synthesis and function of hormones, which are essential for preserving bone health. For instance, smoking has been connected to decreased levels of estrogen in women, which is necessary for bone density.

3. Dysfunctional Absorption of Calcium: Calcium, one of the most important minerals for strong bones, is hampered by smoking. The main building block of bones is calcium, and insufficient absorption of this mineral can reduce bone density.

4. Delayed Fracture Healing: Smoking has been linked to both an increased risk of complications after fractures and delayed fracture healing. This is partially because smoking has detrimental effects on oxygen delivery to tissues and blood circulation.

5. Risk of Fractures Increased: Smokers are more likely to fracture, especially hip fractures. Reduced bone density makes bones more brittle and prone to fractures; poor bone healing can make these risks worse.

6. Inflammation and Oxidative Stress: Smoking increases the body's oxidative stress and inflammatory response. Prolonged inflammation can impede the process of bone remodelling, which is the replacement of old bone tissue with new bone, ultimately resulting in bone loss.

7. Modified Bone Microarchitecture: Smoking has a detrimental effect on the bone tissue's microarchitecture, increasing the risk of bone fractures. Bone strength is further compromised by changes in bone form.

8. Early Menopause Onset: Smokers who are female may go through menopause early, which lowers their estrogen levels. Early menopause can hasten bone loss because estrogen protects bone health.

Smoking Cessation and Bone Health:

1. Enhanced Density of Bones: Reducing tobacco use has been linked to increases in bone density. People who stop smoking may gradually regain more bone mass over time.

2. Decreased Fracture Risk: When smoking cessation is achieved, the risk of fractures declines. The sooner one gives up, the greater the likelihood that the effect on bone health will be minimized.

3. Enhanced Fracture Healing: Giving up smoking encourages enhanced oxygen and blood flow, which can enhance fracture healing and lower problems.

4. Hormonal Restoration: Giving up smoking may result in a return of the hormonal balance, especially women's levels of estrogen, which is good for the health of their bones.

5. Reduced Inflammation: Giving up smoking has a good effect on bone remodelling processes by lowering general inflammation in the body.

Limiting Alcohol Intake

Limiting alcohol intake is important for overall health, especially when following an osteoporosis-friendly diet. Excessive alcohol consumption can negatively impact bone health.

Here are some practical tips to help limit alcohol intake while managing osteoporosis:

1. Set realistic goals:

Establish achievable and realistic goals for reducing alcohol consumption. Gradual changes are often more sustainable than drastic ones.

2. Understand serving sizes:

Be aware of standard serving sizes for different alcoholic beverages. Understanding the amount of alcohol in each serving can help you monitor and control your intake.

3. Choose non-alcoholic alternatives:

Opt for non-alcoholic alternatives to replace alcoholic beverages. Consider mocktails, alcohol-free beer, or sparkling water with a splash of fruit juice.

4. Monitor Portion Sizes:

If you choose to drink alcohol, control portion sizes. Use smaller glasses and avoid oversized servings to moderate your intake.

5. Designate Alcohol-Free Days:

Establish specific days of the week as alcohol-free. This can help create a routine and reduce the overall frequency of alcohol consumption.

6. Stay Hydrated:

Drink water between alcoholic beverages to stay hydrated. Hydration is crucial for overall health and can help pace your drinking.

7. Be Mindful of Cocktails:

Cocktails often contain multiple types of alcohol and mixers, leading to increased calorie and alcohol intake. Choose simpler, lower-alcohol options.

8. Plan Ahead:

Plan your social outings and events with alcohol in mind. Decide in advance how much you'll drink and stick to your plan.

9. Eat Before Drinking:

Consuming a balanced meal before drinking can slow down the absorption of alcohol, reducing its impact on your body.

10. Find Support:

Seek support from friends or family members if you're trying to limit your alcohol intake. Having a support system can make it easier to stick to your goals.

11. Learn to Say No:

Be assertive in declining offers of alcoholic beverages, especially if you're trying to limit your intake. Politely, but firmly, communicate your decision.

12. Educate Yourself:

Understand the impact of alcohol on bone health and overall well-being. Knowledge can be a powerful motivator for making healthier choices.

Sunlight and Vitamin D

Sunlight and vitamin D play crucial roles in bone health and are essential components of an osteoporosis-friendly diet.

While sunshine is a natural source of vitamin D, it's crucial to remember that prolonged sun exposure without adequate protection can raise the risk of skin cancer. Thus, it's critical to strike a balance between getting enough vitamin D and shielding your skin from UV radiation.

Sunlight and Osteoporosis:

1. Vitamin D Synthesis: Exposure to sunlight is the body's natural process of producing vitamin D. Sunlight-induced ultraviolet B (UVB) ray exposure causes the skin to begin producing vitamin D.

2. Calcium Absorption: The small intestine needs vitamin D in order to absorb calcium. It needs adequate absorption of calcium to keep bones strong and dense.

3. Bone Health: By promoting general bone health, sunlight helps prevent osteoporosis. Vitamin D aids in the mineralization of bones by controlling blood levels of phosphorus and calcium.

Diet for Osteoporosis and Vitamin D:

1. Calcium Absorption: Vitamin D improves calcium absorption from food. Eating foods high in calcium and vitamin D guarantees that the calcium that is absorbed is used for bone health.

2. Bone development: By promoting the synthesis of osteocalcin, a protein necessary for bone structure, vitamin D contributes to the development of new bones.

3. Muscle Function: Vitamin D plays a vital role in maintaining muscle function. Strong muscles help maintain bone health and lower the chance of fractures and falls in those who have osteoporosis.

4. Immune System Support: Sufficient amounts of vitamin D maintain a robust immune system, which is critical for general health, including bone health.

Tips for Sunlight Exposure and Vitamin D Intake:

1. Sun Exposure: Try to get moderate amounts of sun exposure, especially in the early morning or late afternoon when the sun's UVB rays are more beneficial for the synthesis of vitamin D.

Depending on your skin tone and geographic area, expose your face, arms, and legs to sunshine for 10 to 30 minutes a few times a week.

2. Dietary Sources of Vitamin D: Include foods high in vitamin D in your diet, such as egg yolks, beef liver, fortified dairy products (milk, yogurt), fatty fish (salmon, mackerel, tuna), and plant-based milk substitutes.

3. Supplements: Vitamin D supplements could be advised if there is little to no sun exposure or inadequate food consumption.

4. Regular Monitoring: Use blood tests to periodically assess vitamin D levels. This guarantees that your levels stay appropriate for the best possible bone health.

5. Balance with Calcium: Make sure you're getting enough calcium and vitamin D in your diet. Together, these two nutrients promote the health of your bones.

CHAPTER SIX

BUILDING AND MAINTAINING BONE DENSITY

Understanding Bone Density Tests

Comprehending the findings of bone density tests is crucial for evaluating the health of bones and spotting possible problems such as osteoporosis. The most widely used test for bone density is known as Dual-Energy X-ray Absorptiometry, or DXA (DEXA).

The results can be interpreted as follows:

T-Score:

1. Normal Bone Density: A T-score greater than -1 is regarded as typical. This indicates that you have a decreased risk of fractures and that your bone density is within the normal range for your age.

2. Osteopenia (Low Bone Mass): A T-score ranging from -1 to -2.5 signifies osteopenia, a medical disease marked by reduced bone density compared to normal. Since this stage is thought to be a prelude to osteoporosis, changing one's lifestyle may be advised to stop additional bone loss.

3. Osteoporosis: An osteoporosis T-score of -2.5 or less is considered to exist. This indicates that your bone density is far lower than normal, which raises the possibility of fractures. At this point, treatment and preventative measures are usually advised.

Z-Score:

1. Within Expected Range: If your Z-score falls within the expected range for your age, it means that the bone density of people in your age group is comparable to yours. Since it compares your bone density to that of individuals of the same age and gender, it is more pertinent to younger people.

2. Below predicted range: If your Z-score is much lower than what is predicted for your age, it could be a symptom of problems including hormone imbalances, long-term illnesses, or drugs that influence bone health. It might be necessary to conduct additional research to find the root causes.

Other Considerations:

1. Fracture Risk: Your doctor may evaluate your total fracture risk based on clinical criteria, such as age, family history, and prior fractures, in addition to T- and Z-scores.

2. Rate of Bone Loss: The pace of bone loss may be assessed by your doctor if you've had several bone density tests over time. This data facilitates comprehension of the evolution of changes in bone density.

3. Individualized Recommendations: Your doctor will evaluate the findings in light of your risk factors and general health. If necessary, they will offer personalized suggestions for medication, lifestyle modifications, and other therapies.

Important Details:

Trends Over Time: Rather than concentrating only on one test result, it's critical to look at patterns in bone density over time. A useful tool for evaluating the success of treatments is change monitoring.

Clinical Assessment: Determining bone density is only one part of determining bone health. Determining the whole picture requires careful consideration of clinical judgment, medical history, and other risk factors.

Medications and Treatments

Several medications and treatments are available for managing osteoporosis. The choice of treatment depends on factors such as the severity of osteoporosis, risk factors, and individual health considerations.

Here are some common medications and treatments for osteoporosis:

Medications:

1. Bisphosphonates: Actonel (Risendronate), Boniva (Ibandronate), Reclast (Zoledronic Acid), Alendronate **(Fosamax):** These drugs aid in decreasing bone loss, boosting bone mass, and lowering the chance of fractures. Usually, they are taken orally or intravenously in the case of zoledronic acid.

2. Raloxifene (Evista):

Selective Estrogen Receptor Modulators (SERMs): In postmenopausal women, raloxifene helps prevent bone loss by mimicking the effects of estrogen. It is especially helpful for people who have previously had breast cancer.

3. HRT (hormone replacement therapy):

Progestin with or without estrogen: Postmenopausal women may be taken HRT to prevent the effects of decreasing estrogen levels on bone density. However, because there could be hazards involved, using HRT must be carefully examined.

4. Calcitonin:

Calcitonin (Miacalcin or Fortical): Women who have gone through menopause and are unable to take other osteoporosis treatments may be offered this hormone, which aids in controlling the body's calcium levels.

5. Denosumab:

Denosumab (Prolia): This drug is an antibody that prevents the resorption of bone. Every six months, an injection is given of it.

6. Teriparatide:

Teriparatide (Forteo): This artificial version of parathyroid hormone promotes the growth of new bone. Usually, people who are at a greater risk of fractures are prescribed it.

7. Abaloparatide:

Abaloparatide (Tymlos): Another medication that works similarly to teriparatide to promote bone growth and density is abaloparatide.

Treatments:

1. Supplements of Calcium and Vitamin D: Sufficient consumption of calcium and vitamin D is necessary for healthy bones. It could be advised to take supplements to make sure people get all the nutrients they need each day.

2. Lifestyle Modifications: Frequent weight-bearing activities can help increase bone density. Examples of these exercises include walking and strength training. Exercises for flexibility and balance lower the chance of falls.

3. Fall Prevention Measures: Reducing the likelihood of falls in the house, utilizing assistive technology, and taking safety measures can all help avoid fractures.

4. Smoking Cessation and Alcohol Moderation: Two crucial lifestyle adjustments to promote general bone health are giving up smoking and consuming less alcohol.

5. Bone Health Monitoring: Frequent bone density testing helps track changes in bone density over time and determine how well a treatment is working.

6. Fracture Management: If fractures occur, fast and adequate medical care is crucial for maximum recovery.

7. Personalized Treatment Programs: Based on variables such as age, gender, general health, and risk factors, treatment programs are frequently customized.

Tips for Long-Term Bone Health

A combination of dietary plans, lifestyle decisions, and preventative actions are necessary to maintain long-term bone health.

To encourage and maintain strong bones throughout life, consider the following advice:

1. Sufficient Consumption of Calcium:

Eat meals high in calcium: To guarantee that you are getting enough calcium, eat dairy products, leafy green vegetables, tofu, almonds, and fortified meals.

2. Optimal Vitamin D levels:

Sun Exposure: To enable your skin to naturally synthesize vitamin D, aim for moderate sun exposure. Sunlight synthesis is affected by age, skin tone, and geographic location, among other factors.

Dietary Sources: Incorporate foods high in vitamin D, such as fortified dairy products, egg yolks, fatty fish, and plant-based substitutes.

3. A Well-Balanced Diet:

Foods Packed with Nutrients: Eat a diet balanced and full of whole grains, fruits, vegetables, lean meats, and healthy fats.

Protein Intake: Since protein is necessary for healthy bones, make sure you consume plenty of it from foods like fish, chicken, beans, and nuts.

4. Getting Regular Exercise:

Weight-Bearing Exercises: To increase bone density, perform weight-bearing exercises like walking, running, dancing, and strength training.

Balance and Flexibility Exercises: Incorporate activities like yoga and tai chi to enhance balance and flexibility, reducing the risk of falls.

5. Lifestyle Choices:

Quit Smoking: Smoking significantly influences bone health. Quitting smoking helps with overall well-being, including bone density.

Reduce Alcohol Intake: Drink in moderation, as too much alcohol might hinder the absorption of calcium and raise the risk of fractures.

6. Preventing Falls:

Home Safety: Reduce the risk of trips and falls by adding grab bars, making sure your home is well-lit, and so on.

Regular Eye Exams: By maintaining healthy eyesight, routine eye exams can lower the risk of falls.

8. Health of Hormones:

Hormone Balance: Preserve hormonal equilibrium, particularly in women who have gone through menopause.

9. Compliance with Medication:

Adhere to Treatment Plans: If medicine is indicated for bone health, follow the suggested course of action.

10. Keep Your Water Up:

Proper Water Consumption: Drink plenty of water to stay hydrated, as it promotes bone health as well as general health.

11. Frequent Medical Exams:

Comprehensive Health Assessments: Routine medical examinations assist in detecting and resolving possible problems that may impact bone health.

12. Youth Bone-Healthy Habits:

Start Early: Promote bone-healthy behaviours throughout infancy and youth. Long-term bone health is influenced by the development of strong bones throughout these crucial times.

CHAPTER SEVEN

OVERCOMING CHALLENGES

Dealing with Dietary Restrictions

Dietary constraints can be difficult to deal with, but a healthy and fulfilling diet can be maintained with careful preparation and inventiveness. These pointers can assist you in navigating dietary limits, regardless of whether they are brought on by allergies, medical issues, or personal preferences:

1. "Aware of Your Limitations"

Read Labels: Acquire the skill of reading food labels to spot possible allergies or ingredients that might be limited.

2. Organize well-balanced meals:

Vibrant Food Selections: To guarantee a balanced and varied diet, try a range of foods that fit your dietary requirements.

Include Nutrient-Rich Foods: Give nutrient-dense foods priority in order to meet your nutritional demands even with dietary constraints.

3. Preparing Meals:

Plan and Prepare Ahead: Make healthy options easily accessible by planning and preparing meals ahead of time, which will lessen the temptation to deviate from recommended dietary intake.

Batch Cooking: Batch cooking guarantees that you always have meals that comply with regulations and can save you time.

4. Survey Other Ingredients:

Substitute Ingredients: Find and utilize alternatives to ingredients that are banned. For instance, people who are gluten-intolerant can use almond flour instead of wheat flour for baking.

Try New Foods: To add diversity to your diet, experiment with different grains, flours, and plant-based proteins.

5. Become Informed:

Learn Cooking Techniques: Develop the knowledge and abilities to prepare meals that maximize the ingredients that fit your constraints.

Stay Informed: Discover new items and recipes that meet your dietary needs.

6. Introduction:

Inform Others: Make sure the staff at the restaurant, your loved ones, and friends are aware of your dietary limitations and are able to meet them.

To ensure you have something to eat during parties,

Be Proactive: Offer to bring a meal that fits your dietary restrictions.

7. Community Aid:

Connect with Others: Visit websites or support groups where people with comparable challenges exchange stories, advice, and recipes.

Inform your loved ones and friends about your food restrictions so they can offer you support and understanding.

9. Conscious Dining:

Pay Attention to Your Body: Keep an eye on how your body reacts to various foods. This might assist you in customizing your diet to meet your specific demands.

Savor the Experience: Rather than concentrating on your dietary constraints, concentrate on the tastes and sensations of the items you can eat.

10. Maintain an optimistic outlook:

Pay Attention to What You Can Eat: Focus on the quantity of items that meet your nutritional needs rather than the constraints.

Celebrate Little Victories: Honor and celebrate any accomplishments, no matter how minor, related to sticking to your diet plan.

Staying Motivated with Exercise

Maintaining bone health requires exercise motivation, which can be difficult when controlling osteoporosis with a certain diet. The following advice can help you maintain your motivation and consistency when exercising:

1. Achieve realistic objectives:

Fitness Goals, Both Short- and Long-Term:

- Specify your long- and short-term objectives. These may have to do with general fitness, bone health, or particular exercises.

Measurable and Specific Objectives:

- Specify and quantify your objectives. For instance, set goals like walking a certain distance, doing a certain amount of reps, or strengthening up to a certain degree.

2. Discover Fun Activities:

Select Your Favorite Activities: Take part in enjoyable exercises. The more activities you enjoy, whether it's dancing, hiking, swimming, or weightlifting, the more likely you are to remain with them.

Variety: Add a range of workouts to your regimen to keep it fresh. This works several muscle areas and keeps you from becoming bored.

3. Establish a Routine:

Regular Timetable: Create a workout regimen that works with your everyday schedule. To create a habit, one must remain consistent.

Make it Non-Negotiable: Treat your workouts, like any other significant obligation, as non-negotiable parts of your day.

4. Include Third Parties:

Find an Exercise Partner: Locate a buddy or relative to work out with. Exercise can be more pleasurable and motivating when done with a partner.

Join Classes or Groups: Take part in fitness courses or gatherings. This fosters a feeling of solidarity and community.

5. Monitor Your Development:

Maintain a Journal: To monitor your improvement, keep a journal of your workouts. Honor accomplishments, no matter how modest, to increase drive.

Use Fitness Apps: Look into fitness applications that can assist you in keeping track of your exercises, establishing objectives, and giving you a sense of success.

6. Adjust Workouts Safely:

Gradual Progression: Begin with workouts appropriate for your current level of fitness and advance progressively. To avoid being hurt, don't overexert yourself.

7. Make it Fun:

Incorporate music or podcasts: To make your workout more fun, listen to music or podcasts. This can help you forget about your discomfort and accelerate the passage of time.

Activities Outside: Make the most of outside activities. In the great outdoors, riding, hiking, and walking can offer a welcome change of pace.

8. Give yourself a reward:

Celebrate Milestones: Honor your achievements in terms of fitness. When you reach a certain objective, treat yourself to a well-deserved reward.

Positive Reinforcement: Pay attention to the good things that happen to you when you exercise regularly, such as better mood, more energy, or better sleep.

9. Become Informed:

Know the Advantages: Acquire knowledge of the particular advantages of exercise for osteoporosis and bone health. Gaining insight into the effects can inspire even more.

10. Adjust as Required:

Be Flexible: Adjust your workout schedule as needed. Because life can be unpredictable, it's acceptable to modify your exercise regimen as necessary.

Coping with Osteoporosis Emotionally

Adapting to a chronic health condition that may affect multiple facets of your life can be emotionally taxing while dealing with osteoporosis. The following are some coping mechanisms to help you deal with osteoporosis emotionally:

1. Acknowledge and understand your emotions.

Identify Emotions: Accept any feelings you could be going through, such as fear, annoyance, or melancholy. Coping begins with accepting these feelings.

Educate Yourself: Gain a better understanding of osteoporosis by learning more about the condition. Having knowledge gives you the ability to take charge of your health and make wise decisions.

2. Create a Support Network:

Convey to Special Someone: Share your feelings with your family and friends. Expressing your ideas might promote understanding and emotional support.

4. Pay Attention to What You Can Control:

Make healthy lifestyle choices. Accept lifestyle modifications that enhance general wellbeing. This includes maintaining a healthy diet, getting regular exercise, and abstaining from bad behaviors like smoking and binge drinking.

Medication Adherence: Comply with your treatment plan if you are prescribed medication. It can give you a sense of control to know that you are making efforts to manage your illness.

5. Control Your Stress:

Apply Stress-Reduction Techniques: Take part in stress-reduction exercises like yoga, mindfulness, meditation, or deep breathing. Reducing stress enhances general wellbeing.

Activities and Hobbies: Take up interests and pastimes that make you happy and calm. Spending time on interesting activities can serve as a useful diversion.

7. Achieve realistic goals:

Accept Limitations: Recognize and accept your physical limitations while keeping your attention on your remaining goals. Having reasonable expectations will help you deal with disappointment.

Celebrate Achievements: Honor minor victories in maintaining your well-being or following your treatment regimen. Acknowledging any achievement, no matter how small, improves spirits.

8. Stay Positive:

Optimistic Mentality:

- Develop an optimistic outlook. To cultivate a more positive attitude, pay attention to the parts of life that make you happy and grateful.

Humor and Laughter: Make humor and laughter a part of your everyday existence. It is commonly recognized that laughter improves mood and general wellbeing.

10. Plan for the Future:

Set Goals: Establish realistic goals for the future. These could be related to your health, personal development, or fun events.

Financial Planning: Take into account budgeting for prospective medical expenses. Feeling secure comes from knowing you have a plan in place.

CONCLUSION

In summary, "Osteoporosis Diet and Exercises" provides a thorough and approachable manual for anybody attempting to understand the nuances of osteoporosis. With thirty years of experience, our prestigious publishing firm is proud to offer a multitude of information to enable readers to effectively manage this bone health condition.

The book explores the complex interactions that occur between overall lifestyle choices, exercise, and diet to strengthen bones and lessen the effects of osteoporosis. Readers are guided through important themes, including understanding osteoporosis, nutritional considerations, exercise routines, and useful recommendations for everyday living, by the well-crafted table of contents, which offers an organized approach.

The book guarantees a complete explanation of osteoporosis by going over its description, causes, and risk factors, as well as its indications and symptoms. It goes even beyond explaining the critical function that meals, nutritional supplements, and other necessary components have in building healthy bones, laying a solid foundation for the parts that follow.

The book's pragmatism is evident in its suggestions for meal planning, creating diets that are specific to each person, and creating foods that support bone health. A holistic approach is shown in the emphasis on grocery shopping guidelines, which acknowledge the significance of lifestyle decisions made outside of the kitchen.

Regarding exercise, the book offers a thorough examination of numerous exercises that are good for osteoporosis, along with advice on how to design safe and efficient workout regimens. Recognizing the dynamic nature of bone health, weight-bearing and resistance exercises combine to provide a well-rounded approach to physical activity.

In addition to the physiological components, the book discusses lifestyle changes that have an impact on osteoporosis, such as quitting smoking and consuming alcohol in moderation. It explores the psychological difficulties associated with managing osteoporosis on an emotional level, identifies them, and provides solutions.

The book's dedication to providing a comprehensive resource is demonstrated by the inclusion of drugs, therapies, and long-term methods for bone health. It encourages readers to manage osteoporosis with knowledge, involvement, and initiative, advocating for a proactive approach to healthcare.

In the end, "Osteoporosis Diet and Exercises" serves as a traveling companion for achieving ideal bone health rather than just a book. It is the ideal combination of scientific knowledge, useful guidance, and inspirational writing, and it is proof of our dedication to providing high-quality information that enables people to take control of their health and wellbeing. Readers will leave this illuminating and motivating trip with the skills and information necessary to manage osteoporosis gracefully and with resiliency.